PREMATURE GREYING

Science, Solutions, and Self-Discovery

Dr Mukesh Aggarwal

CONTENTS

UNDERSTANDING PREMATURE GREYING

Introduction

Premature greying refers to the early onset of grey or white hair, often before the age of 20 or in one's 20s. Genetics play a significant role, but other factors like stress, nutritional deficiencies, certain medical conditions, and lifestyle choices can contribute to premature greying. It occurs due to a decrease in melanin production, the pigment responsible for hair color, resulting in the hair appearing grey or white.

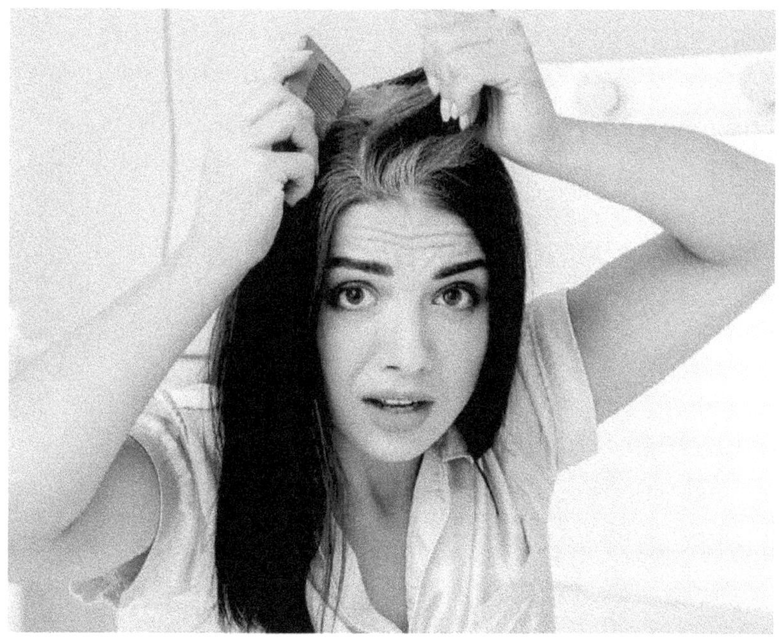

Differentiating between normal and premature greying

Greying of hair is a natural phenomenon that usually occurs with age as the body's production of melanin, the pigment responsible for hair color, decreases. However, in some cases, this process happens earlier than expected, leading to premature greying. Understanding the differences between normal and premature greying is crucial to address concerns and take appropriate steps.

Normal greying of hair typically begins in one's 30s or 40s, progressing gradually over time. It is primarily influenced by genetics and is considered a part of the natural aging process. As individuals age, the melanocytes, cells responsible for producing melanin, gradually decline in function, leading to a decrease in pigment production. As a result, hair loses its color and turns grey or white.

On the other hand, premature greying occurs at a younger age, often before 20 or in one's 20s, and progresses at a faster rate than normal greying. Genetics still play a role, but other factors such as stress, nutritional deficiencies, hormonal changes, certain medical conditions (like thyroid disorders or vitiligo), smoking, and environmental factors can contribute significantly to premature greying. These factors can interfere with melanin production, causing hair to lose its color prematurely.

Distinguishing between the two types of greying involves considering various factors. Normal greying typically starts at a later age, progresses slowly, and is mostly determined by genetics. In contrast, premature greying is characterized by an early onset, rapid progression, and can be influenced by lifestyle, health, and environmental factors.

Addressing premature greying involves adopting strategies to slow down or manage the process. Lifestyle changes such as reducing stress, maintaining a balanced diet rich in vitamins and minerals, quitting smoking, and using hair care products that promote melanin production or cover greys can help manage premature greying. Consulting a healthcare professional or a dermatologist can also provide insights into underlying health conditions contributing to premature greying and appropriate treatment options.

In conclusion, while greying of hair is a natural part of aging, premature greying occurs earlier than usual and involves various factors beyond genetics. Recognizing the differences between normal and premature greying is essential to address concerns effectively and take necessary steps to manage or treat premature greying based on its underlying causes.

Genetic and environmental factors influencing premature greying

Premature greying, the early onset of grey or white hair before the typical age, is influenced by a combination of genetic and environmental factors. While genetics play a significant role in determining hair color and its changes, various environmental elements can also contribute to the premature greying process.

Genetic factors have a considerable impact on premature greying. The inheritance of genes associated with melanin production and distribution determines the onset and progression of greying. Variations in genes responsible for regulating melanocytes, the cells producing melanin, can affect the rate at which hair loses its pigment. Research has shown that individuals with a family history of premature greying are more likely to experience it themselves, indicating a strong genetic component.

However, environmental factors also play a crucial role in premature greying. Stress, both physical and emotional, can accelerate the greying process. Chronic stress can lead to an increase in the production of free radicals, which can damage melanocytes and impede melanin production. Lifestyle choices such as smoking and an unhealthy diet lacking essential vitamins and minerals like B vitamins, iron, copper, and antioxidants can also contribute to premature greying by impacting melanin synthesis.

Furthermore, certain medical conditions can trigger premature greying. Thyroid disorders, vitiligo, autoimmune diseases, and deficiencies in vitamin B12 have been linked to early greying. Additionally, exposure to environmental pollutants, ultraviolet (UV) radiation, and chemicals in hair care products can damage hair follicles and affect melanin production, leading to premature greying.

Understanding the interplay between genetic predispositions and environmental influences is vital in managing premature greying. While genetics establish the baseline for greying, environmental factors can either hasten or delay this process. Adopting a healthy lifestyle, managing stress effectively, consuming a balanced diet rich in essential nutrients, and protecting hair from environmental damage can help slow down or manage premature greying.

In conclusion, premature greying is influenced by a complex interplay between genetic predispositions and environmental factors. While genetics lay the groundwork for the onset and progression of greying, environmental elements such as stress, lifestyle choices, medical conditions, and exposure to pollutants can significantly impact the timing and pace of premature greying. Understanding these influences is crucial in developing strategies to manage or slow down the premature greying process effectively.

THE SCIENCE BEHIND PREMATURE GREYING

Premature graying is often influenced by genetics, stress, and lifestyle factors. It's primarily due to a decline in melanin production, the pigment responsible for hair color. Genetics play a significant role, but stress, nutritional deficiencies, smoking, and certain medical conditions can also contribute to early graying by impacting melanocytes, the cells producing melanin.

Mechanisms and causes of premature greying

Premature graying of hair, also known as canities, is a multifaceted process influenced by various mechanisms and causes. While it's commonly associated with aging, its onset before the age of 20-30 is considered premature.

Mechanisms:

1. Melanin Production Decline: The primary cause of hair color is melanin, produced by melanocytes within hair follicles. As individuals age, melanocyte activity decreases, leading to less pigment production and, subsequently, gray or white hair.

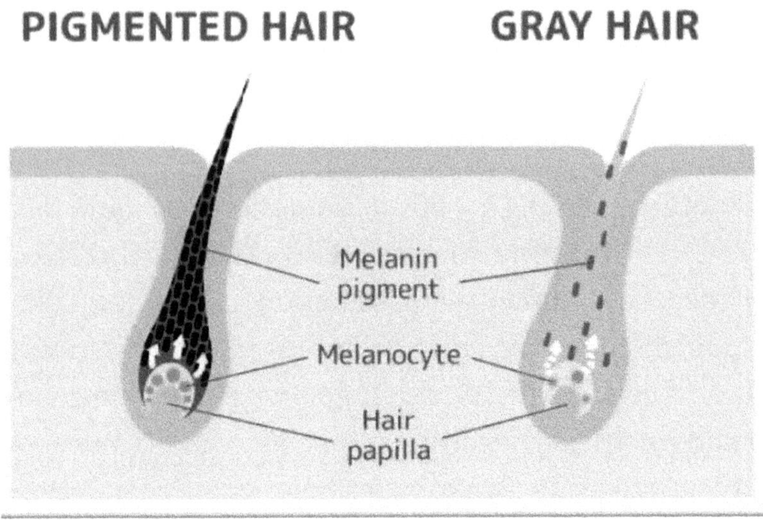

2. Genetics: Genetic predisposition is a significant factor. Certain genes can determine when and how quickly graying occurs. If your parents experienced premature graying, you're more likely to encounter it too.

3. Oxidative Stress: Accumulation of reactive oxygen species (ROS) due to factors like stress, pollution, and UV radiation can damage melanocytes, hastening the graying process.

4. Autoimmune Conditions: Conditions like vitiligo, where the body attacks its pigment-producing cells, can cause premature graying in affected areas.

Causes:

1. Stress: Chronic stress elevates cortisol levels, affecting melanocyte function and leading to premature graying.

2. Lifestyle Factors: Unhealthy habits like smoking, poor diet lacking essential nutrients (vitamins B12, D, E, and minerals like copper), and inadequate sleep contribute to premature graying.

3. Medical Conditions: Thyroid disorders, anemia, and certain other medical conditions can interfere with melanin production, resulting in early graying.
4. Chemical Exposure: Exposure to harsh chemicals in hair products or frequent use of hair dyes may accelerate graying.

Understanding these mechanisms and causes helps in adopting preventive measures. Managing stress, maintaining a balanced diet rich in vitamins and minerals, avoiding harmful chemicals, and seeking medical advice for underlying health conditions can help delay premature graying and promote healthier hair.

Role of genetics and hereditary factors

Genetics and hereditary factors play pivotal roles in shaping various aspects of our lives, influencing everything from physical traits to predispositions for certain diseases. The intricate interplay of genes inherited from our parents determines a significant portion of who we are.

Role of Genetics:

1. Physical Traits: Genes dictate traits like eye color, hair texture, height, and facial features. Dominant and recessive genes from parents blend to create unique combinations in offspring.

2. Predisposition to Diseases: Genetic factors contribute to susceptibility to various diseases, including heart conditions, diabetes, certain cancers, and genetic disorders like cystic fibrosis or sickle cell anemia.

3. Metabolism and Health: Genes influence metabolism, impacting how efficiently our bodies process food and nutrients, potentially affecting weight and overall health.

Hereditary Factors:

1. Inheritance Patterns: Traits are passed down through generations following specific inheritance patterns, such as dominant, recessive, or polygenic inheritance.

2. Family History: A family's medical history provides insights into inherited conditions or susceptibilities, aiding in understanding potential health risks.

3. Epigenetics: Beyond DNA sequences, environmental factors can modify gene expression without altering the DNA sequence itself, affecting how genes are turned on or off, potentially impacting future generations.

Impact on Personal and Medical Decisions:

Understanding genetic predispositions can inform personal choices and medical decisions. Genetic testing helps identify risks for certain diseases, allowing proactive measures for prevention or early detection. In reproductive planning, knowledge of inherited conditions aids in informed family planning decisions.

Conclusion:

Genetics and hereditary factors form the blueprint of our existence, influencing not only physical traits but also health outcomes and susceptibilities. While genetics lay the groundwork, environmental factors also significantly shape our lives. The combination of both genetics and environment defines who we are and how we navigate our health and wellbeing. Continued research in genetics promises further insights into understanding and managing various facets of our lives.

Oxidative stress and its impact on premature greying

Oxidative stress, caused by an imbalance between antioxidants and free radicals in the body, significantly impacts premature greying. Here's how:
Mechanism:

1. Melanocyte Damage: Oxidative stress triggers an excess production of free radicals. These unstable molecules can damage cells, including melanocytes responsible for producing melanin (hair pigment). When melanocytes are affected, they produce less melanin, leading to gray or white hair.

2. Accelerated Aging: Oxidative stress accelerates aging processes, including those affecting hair follicles. As a result, hair prematurely loses its natural color due to diminished melanin production.

Factors Contributing to Oxidative Stress:

1. Environmental Factors: Exposure to pollutants, UV radiation, and toxins from the environment contributes to oxidative stress, impacting the hair follicles and leading to premature graying.

2. Lifestyle Choices: Unhealthy habits like smoking, poor diet, lack of exercise, and high stress levels increase oxidative stress in the body, potentially hastening the onset of premature graying.

Mitigation and Prevention:

1. Antioxidants: Consuming a diet rich in antioxidants (found in fruits, vegetables, nuts, and seeds) helps neutralize free radicals, reducing oxidative stress and potentially slowing down premature graying.

2. Lifestyle Changes: Adopting a healthy lifestyle by managing stress, quitting smoking, and minimizing exposure to environmental pollutants can mitigate oxidative stress and its impact on hair health.

Understanding the relationship between oxidative stress and premature greying emphasizes the importance of lifestyle choices and antioxidant-rich diets in maintaining healthy hair and potentially delaying the onset of gray hair.

Chapter 3

LIFESTYLE AND ENVIRONMENTAL TRIGGERS

Premature greying can result from various factors like genetics, stress, nutritional deficiencies, and certain medical conditions. Lifestyle choices such as smoking, excessive stress, poor diet, and environmental factors like pollution might contribute too. While genetics play a significant role, maintaining a healthy lifestyle with a balanced diet and stress management could help slow down premature greying.

Stress and its relation to premature greying

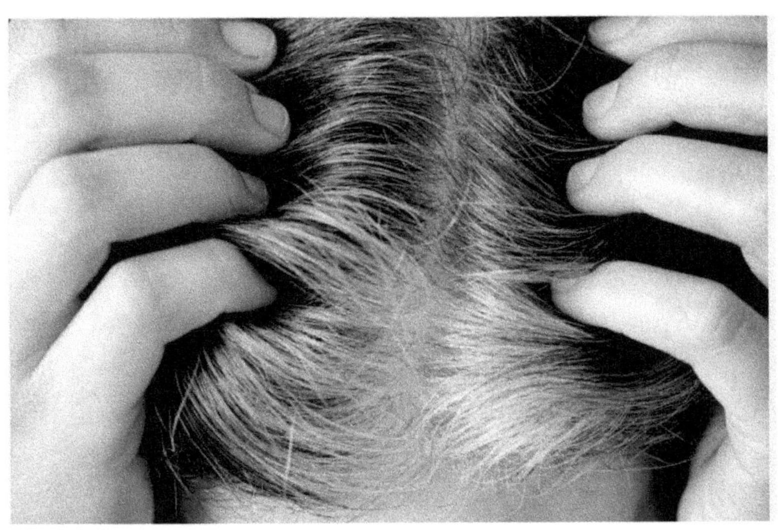

Premature greying, often attributed to genetics, can also have links to stress. Stress triggers the release of hormones like cortisol, impacting the body's melanocytes responsible for hair pigmentation. When stress disrupts these cells, it can accelerate the greying process.

The connection between stress and premature greying has gained attention in recent years. Chronic stress, due to work, personal life, or other factors, can impact various bodily functions, including hair health. While it's not the sole cause, stress management through mindfulness, meditation, exercise, and a balanced lifestyle can potentially mitigate premature greying. Understanding and addressing stress are crucial not only for mental health but also for maintaining overall well-being, potentially impacting hair health and greying.

Dietary factors affecting hair pigmentation

Dietary factors play a pivotal role in maintaining healthy hair pigmentation. Nutrients like vitamins (especially B vitamins like Biotin, B12, and Folate), minerals (such as iron, copper, zinc), and proteins are essential for the synthesis of melanin, the pigment responsible for hair color.

A deficiency in these nutrients can lead to impaired melanin production, potentially accelerating the onset of premature greying. For instance, inadequate intake of B vitamins affects melanin production, while deficiencies in minerals like iron and copper disrupt the enzymes involved in pigment synthesis.

Moreover, antioxidants like vitamins A, C, and E protect hair follicles from oxidative stress, preserving hair color. Including a balanced diet rich in leafy greens, nuts, seeds, fish, lean meats, and fruits helps ensure a sufficient intake of these vital nutrients, promoting healthy hair pigmentation.

While dietary factors are significant, it's essential to note that premature greying can also result from genetics and other non-dietary factors. Nonetheless, maintaining a nutritious diet can contribute to healthier hair and potentially delay premature greying.

Environmental factors: pollution, UV exposure, and their contribution to premature greying

Pollution, particularly air pollution, exposes the hair and scalp to harmful particles and toxins. These pollutants generate oxidative stress, leading to an imbalance in free radicals that damage the hair follicles. Oxidative stress negatively impacts melanocytes, hindering their ability to produce melanin, which results in premature greying.

UV radiation, primarily from the sun, is another environmental factor that can accelerate greying. Prolonged exposure to UV rays damages the hair shaft, weakens the follicles, and disrupts the melanin production process. This exposure induces oxidative stress, causing premature aging of the hair and potentially contributing to premature greying.

To mitigate the effects of environmental factors on premature greying, protective measures like wearing hats or scarves in polluted areas and using hair care products with UV protection can help. Additionally, adopting a healthy hair care routine and consuming antioxidant-rich foods can potentially counteract the oxidative stress caused by pollution and UV exposure, supporting hair health and delaying premature greying.

Chapter 4

MANAGING PREMATURE GREYING

Premature greying can stem from various factors like genetics, stress, diet, or health conditions. Consider these tips: maintain a balanced diet rich in vitamins and minerals, manage stress through meditation or exercise, avoid smoking, and use hair care products designed for your hair type. Consult a healthcare professional for personalized advice.

Hair Care Practices to Mitigate Premature Greying

Hair, often considered a symbol of beauty and vitality, can be affected by premature greying, a condition that can be distressing for many individuals. While genetics play a significant role, adopting specific hair care practices can help mitigate premature greying and maintain healthy hair.

Firstly, a balanced diet plays a crucial role in maintaining hair health. Incorporating foods rich in essential vitamins and minerals like iron, B vitamins (particularly Biotin and B12), zinc, and antioxidants helps nourish the hair follicles and prevents premature greying. Foods such as leafy greens, nuts, eggs, fish, and berries are beneficial in this regard.

Managing stress is another pivotal factor in preventing premature greying. Chronic stress can accelerate the greying process. Engaging in stress-relieving activities such as yoga, meditation, or regular exercise can help reduce stress levels, thereby positively impacting hair health.

Furthermore, proper hair care routines are essential. Gentle handling of hair, avoiding excessive heat styling, and using mild, sulfate-free shampoos can prevent damage to the hair shafts, reducing the likelihood of premature greying. Additionally, regular conditioning and deep conditioning treatments can help maintain hair moisture and prevent brittleness, a common issue associated with premature greying.

Choosing hair care products specifically formulated to target premature greying can also make a difference. Products containing ingredients like antioxidants, keratin, and peptides can help strengthen hair, delay greying, and promote overall hair health.

Protecting hair from environmental damage is equally crucial. UV rays, pollution, and harsh weather conditions can damage hair follicles, leading to premature greying. Wearing hats or scarves when exposed to the sun and using protective hair products can shield hair from environmental stressors.

In conclusion, while premature greying might be influenced by genetic factors beyond our control, adopting a holistic approach to hair care practices can significantly mitigate its effects. A balanced diet, stress management, gentle hair care routines, and using appropriate hair care products are key elements in maintaining healthy hair and delaying premature greying.

By incorporating these practices into daily life, individuals can embrace healthier hair and potentially slow down the onset of premature greying, enhancing not only their appearance but also their confidence and overall well-being.

Medical Treatments for Premature Greying

Premature greying, the early onset of grey or white hair, can be a source of concern for many individuals. While it is primarily influenced by genetics and aging, certain medical treatments and interventions can help manage and potentially reverse this condition to some extent.

One of the primary medical treatments for premature greying involves the use of medications or supplements aimed at addressing nutritional deficiencies. Deficiencies in vitamins such as Biotin, B12, and minerals like iron and copper can contribute to premature greying. Supplements prescribed by healthcare professionals can help balance these deficiencies, potentially slowing down the greying process.

Another approach involves the use of topical solutions or serums containing peptides, antioxidants, and other hair-stimulating agents. These formulations are designed to strengthen hair follicles, improve melanin production, and potentially delay or reverse premature greying.

Furthermore, certain prescription medications used for other conditions, such as autoimmune disorders, have shown incidental effects on hair pigmentation. However, these medications are typically prescribed for their primary purpose, and their impact on greying hair might vary from person to person.

Additionally, newer treatments like photo biomodulation therapy (low-level laser therapy) have emerged as potential options for hair-related issues, including premature greying. These therapies aim to stimulate hair follicles, promoting healthier hair growth and potentially slowing down the greying process.

It's essential to note that while these medical treatments offer possibilities in managing premature greying, their efficacy can vary among individuals. Consulting with a dermatologist or a healthcare professional specializing in hair-related concerns is crucial to determine the most suitable treatment plan based on individual factors like overall health, the cause of premature greying, and other underlying conditions.

In conclusion, medical treatments for premature greying focus on addressing nutritional deficiencies, stimulating hair follicles, and exploring innovative therapies. While these treatments offer promising avenues, more research is needed to ascertain their long-term effectiveness and suitability for different individuals. Seeking professional guidance and understanding the underlying causes are essential steps toward managing premature greying effectively.

Ayurvedic Approach to Treating Premature Greying

Ayurveda, an ancient Indian holistic healing system, offers a unique perspective and natural remedies for various health concerns, including premature greying of hair. According to Ayurveda, premature greying is often attributed to an imbalance in the body's doshas (Vata, Pitta, and Kapha) and can be addressed through a combination of dietary changes, lifestyle modifications, and herbal treatments.

Firstly, Ayurveda emphasizes the importance of maintaining a balanced diet to nurture hair health. Foods such as sesame seeds, curry leaves, Indian gooseberry (amla), nuts, ghee, and certain herbs like Brahmi and Bhringraj are believed to nourish the hair follicles, promote hair pigmentation, and slow down premature greying.

Ayurvedic practitioners often recommend specific lifestyle modifications to manage premature greying. This includes practicing yoga, meditation, and pranayama (breathing exercises) to reduce stress levels, as excessive stress is considered a contributing factor to premature greying in Ayurveda.

Moreover, Ayurvedic treatments often involve the use of herbal remedies and oils. Applying herbal oils like coconut oil infused with Bhringraj, Amla, or Brahmi is a common practice to nurture the scalp, strengthen hair roots, and stimulate melanin production, thereby potentially delaying or reversing premature greying.

Additionally, Ayurvedic formulations such as herbal pastes or powders (like Triphala, Neem, or Shikakai) are used in hair masks or washes to cleanse the scalp, improve blood circulation, and promote overall hair health. These natural ingredients are believed to have properties that support hair pigmentation and prevent premature greying.

Ayurvedic therapies like Shirodhara (continuous pouring of herbal oils on the forehead) and Nasya (nasal administration of herbal oils) are also sometimes recommended to balance the doshas and support overall well-being, which indirectly influences hair health.

However, it's essential to approach Ayurvedic treatments with caution and under the guidance of a qualified Ayurvedic practitioner. Individual responses to herbal remedies may vary, and understanding one's body constitution (prakriti) and specific imbalances is crucial for personalized treatment.

In conclusion, Ayurveda offers a holistic approach to treating premature greying by focusing on dietary adjustments, lifestyle modifications, and the use of natural herbal remedies. While these treatments are generally regarded as safe, consulting an Ayurvedic professional ensures the most appropriate and personalized approach to address premature greying while embracing the holistic principles of Ayurveda.

Home Remedies for Managing Premature Greying

The premature greying of hair can be a source of concern for many individuals, prompting exploration of natural and home-based remedies to mitigate this condition. While genetics play a significant role, incorporating certain home remedies into one's routine can potentially slow down the greying process and support healthier hair.

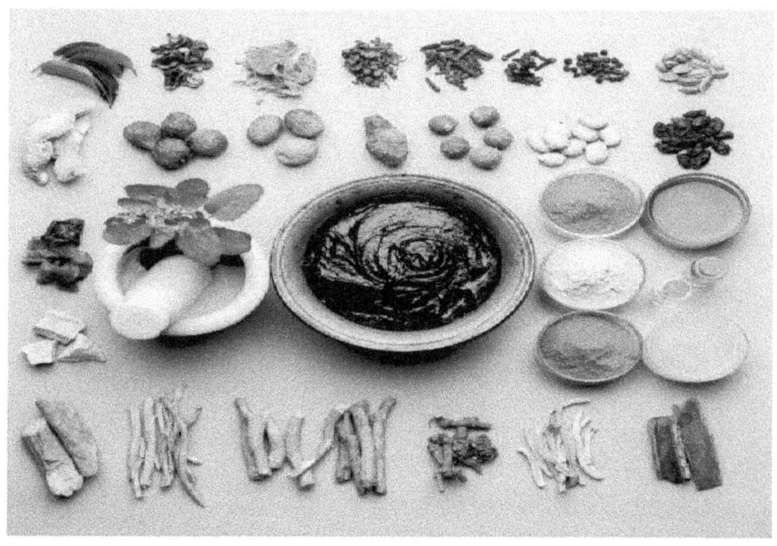

1. Amla (Indian Gooseberry): Amla, renowned for its high vitamin C content and antioxidant properties, is a popular remedy in preventing premature greying. Consuming amla juice or applying amla oil to the scalp is believed to nourish hair follicles, strengthen hair strands, and promote melanin production.

2. Coconut Oil and Curry Leaves: Boiling curry leaves in coconut oil and applying this mixture onto the scalp helps in retaining natural hair pigment. Curry leaves are rich in antioxidants and vitamins essential for hair health, potentially slowing down premature greying.

3. Onion Juice: Onion juice is considered beneficial for its enzyme catalase, which aids in restoring hair's natural color. Applying onion juice to the scalp, though pungent in smell, may help counter premature greying.

4. Black Tea or Coffee Rinses: Rinsing hair with black tea or coffee can add natural color and shine to the hair. The tannins present in these beverages might help darken the hair and temporarily cover grey strands.

5. Henna: Henna, a natural dye derived from the Lawsonia inermis plant, has been used for centuries to color hair naturally. Apart from imparting a reddish hue, it can help cover grey hairs effectively.

6. Rosemary and Sage Infusion: Boiling rosemary and sage in water to create an herbal infusion, then applying and massaging it into the scalp, is believed to prevent premature greying by stimulating hair follicles.

While these home remedies are widely practiced and believed to offer benefits in managing premature greying, individual results may vary. Consistency and patience are key when using these remedies, as significant changes might not be immediately noticeable.

It's crucial to remember that while these remedies are natural, they might not suit everyone, and allergic reactions or adverse effects could occur. Performing a patch test before using any new ingredient extensively is recommended, especially for those with sensitive skin or known allergies.

In conclusion, incorporating these home remedies into one's hair care routine may offer a natural approach to managing premature greying. While these remedies may not completely reverse the process, they can potentially slow down greying, support healthier hair, and serve as an adjunct to overall hair care practices. Seeking professional advice is advisable, especially for those with specific allergies or medical conditions, to ensure the safety and efficacy of these home remedies.

Cosmetic Treatments for Managing Premature Greying

Premature greying, the untimely loss of natural hair pigmentation, can cause distress for individuals seeking to retain their youthful appearance. While primarily influenced by genetics, lifestyle factors, and age, various cosmetic treatments offer solutions to mask or delay the appearance of grey hair.

1. Hair Dyes and Colorants: Hair dyes are the most common cosmetic solution for covering grey hair. They contain chemicals that penetrate the hair shaft to alter its color. Temporary dyes wash out gradually, while semi-permanent and permanent dyes provide longer-lasting coverage. These products offer a wide range of colors to match natural hair shades and provide effective coverage of grey hair.

2. Root Touch-Up Products: These products are designed to camouflage the appearance of grey roots between dyeing sessions. Root touch-up sprays, powders, or mascaras offer a quick fix, concealing grey roots until the next hair coloring session.

3. Hair Mascara and Chalks: Hair mascaras and chalks are temporary solutions that allow individuals to conceal grey strands selectively. These products are applied directly onto the grey areas and can be washed out easily, offering a temporary cover for specific occasions.

4. Highlights and Lowlights: Adding highlights or lowlights to the hair can blend grey strands with the natural hair color, creating dimension and minimizing the stark contrast between grey and pigmented hair.

5. Hair Treatments with Optical Effects: Some hair care products contain light-reflecting particles or polymers that create an optical illusion, reducing the prominence of grey hair by adding shine and enhancing the hair's appearance.

6. Scalp Micropigmentation: This technique involves tattooing the scalp with pigments to simulate the appearance of a closely shaved head of hair, effectively camouflaging areas of grey or thinning hair.

While these cosmetic treatments offer effective methods to mask or delay the appearance of grey hair, it's essential to consider their limitations and potential side effects. Hair dyes and colorants contain chemicals that might cause allergic reactions or damage the hair with frequent use. Additionally, maintaining colored hair requires regular touch-ups to prevent noticeable regrowth.

Choosing the right product and shade that matches the natural hair color, performing patch tests, and following instructions diligently are crucial for minimizing adverse effects.

In conclusion, cosmetic treatments for premature greying provide a range of options for individuals seeking to conceal or delay the appearance of grey hair. While these solutions offer effective means to address aesthetic concerns, they require regular maintenance and careful consideration to ensure safety and minimize potential damage to the hair and scalp. Consulting with hair care professionals or dermatologists can help individuals make informed decisions regarding the most suitable cosmetic treatments for managing premature greying.

Lifestyle changes to slow down or prevent premature greying

Making certain lifestyle changes can potentially slow down or prevent premature greying. Here are some adjustments that might help:

1. Balanced Diet: Ensure your diet includes nutrients essential for hair health, such as vitamins (especially Biotin, B12), minerals (like copper and zinc), and antioxidants. Foods like leafy greens, nuts, seeds, fish, eggs, and fruits contribute to healthier hair.

2. Stress Management: Chronic stress can accelerate premature greying. Practice stress-relieving activities like yoga, meditation, or mindfulness to manage stress levels and potentially slow down the greying process.

3. Quit Smoking: Smoking has been linked to premature greying. Quitting smoking not only benefits overall health but might also positively impact hair health and delay greying.

4. Gentle Hair Care: Avoid harsh hair treatments, excessive heat styling, and tight hairstyles that can damage hair follicles. Use mild, sulfate-free shampoos and conditioners suitable for your hair type.

5. Adequate Hydration: Drinking enough water helps maintain hair hydration and overall health, potentially preventing premature greying.

6. UV Protection: Protect hair from excessive sun exposure by wearing hats or using products with UV protection to prevent damage to hair follicles.

7. Regular Exercise: Engage in regular physical activity to improve blood circulation, which supports hair follicles and overall hair health.

While these lifestyle changes might not completely prevent premature greying, they can contribute to healthier hair and potentially slow down the process. It's essential to consult a healthcare professional or dermatologist for personalized advice on managing premature greying.

PSYCHOLOGICAL AND SOCIAL IMPACTS

Premature greying can have psychological impacts, affecting self-esteem and confidence, especially in younger individuals. Socially, it might lead to feelings of being judged or self-consciousness due to societal beauty standards. Counseling and support can help individuals navigate these challenges and embrace their natural appearance.

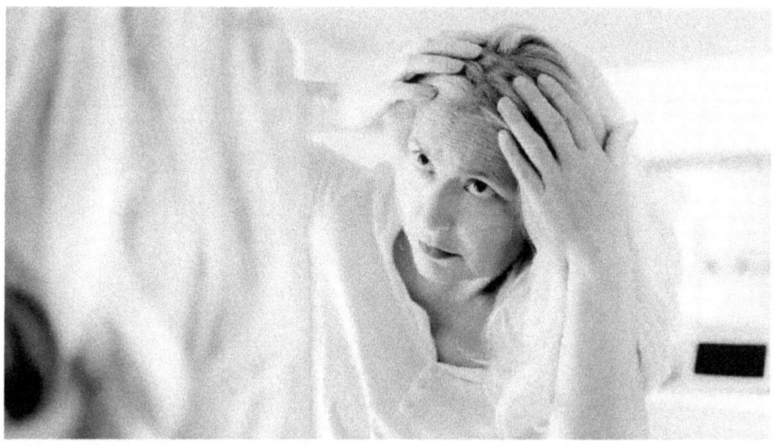

Emotional effects of premature greying

Premature greying, often seen as a cosmetic concern, carries emotional weight that transcends physical appearance. Its psychological impact can be profound, affecting one's self-image, confidence, and emotional well-being.

Firstly, premature greying can trigger a range of emotional responses. For some, it's a stark reminder of aging, causing distress and anxiety about losing youthfulness prematurely. This abrupt change can lead to feelings of shock, disbelief, or even denial, altering one's perception of their own identity.

Secondly, societal norms and beauty standards exacerbate the emotional toll of premature greying. Our culture often associates youthfulness with attractiveness, and grey hair at a young age might create feelings of being unattractive or less desirable. This can contribute to a loss of confidence and self-worth, impacting social interactions and relationships.

Moreover, the emotional effects of premature greying can manifest in various ways. Some individuals might experience heightened self-consciousness, withdrawing from social situations to avoid judgment or uncomfortable scrutiny. Others might grapple with lowered self-esteem, feeling a sense of loss or insecurity about their appearance.

Addressing these emotional impacts involves a multifaceted approach. Encouraging self-acceptance and fostering a positive self-image are crucial. Providing emotional support, whether through therapy, support groups, or open conversations, can help individuals navigate these complex emotions and build resilience.

Furthermore, promoting inclusivity and challenging societal beauty standards can contribute to a more accepting environment for individuals with premature greying. Emphasizing diverse representations of beauty in media and highlighting the naturalness of grey hair can aid in reducing the stigma attached to premature greying.

In conclusion, the emotional effects of premature greying extend far beyond aesthetics. Acknowledging and addressing these emotional impacts is essential for fostering acceptance, self-confidence, and a more inclusive society that values individuality beyond conventional standards of beauty.

Societal perceptions and coping strategies for a premature patient

Societal perceptions of premature greying often revolve around superficial judgments and stereotypes, creating challenges for those affected. Coping strategies are crucial for individuals facing societal scrutiny due to their premature greying.

Firstly, societal perceptions of premature greying can be harsh, as grey hair is typically associated with aging. This can lead to assumptions about a person's age, competence, or even their health. Such perceptions may trigger feelings of insecurity, leading individuals to feel misunderstood or unfairly judged by others.

One coping strategy involves education and awareness. Providing accurate information about premature greying can help dispel myths and misconceptions. By understanding the biological factors contributing to premature greying, society can shift towards a more empathetic and informed view, reducing stigma and discrimination.

Secondly, fostering self-acceptance is vital. Encouraging individuals to embrace their natural appearance and find confidence in their unique features can be empowering. Building resilience and a positive self-image through self-care practices, such as self-affirmation and seeking support from friends, family, or support groups, can aid in navigating societal perceptions.

Additionally, advocating for inclusivity and diversity in beauty standards is essential. Promoting representation of diverse appearances in media and challenging the notion that youth equates to beauty can reshape societal attitudes towards premature greying. Celebrating different forms of beauty helps create an environment that values individuality and uniqueness.

Moreover, communication and openness play a significant role. Encouraging open discussions about premature greying can create a supportive environment where individuals feel comfortable expressing their feelings and experiences. This can foster understanding and empathy, leading to a more inclusive and accepting society.

In conclusion, societal perceptions of premature greying often stem from misconceptions and stereotypes. By employing coping strategies such as education, self-acceptance, advocacy for inclusivity, and open communication, individuals affected by premature greying can navigate societal challenges more effectively. Ultimately, promoting acceptance and understanding can contribute to a more empathetic and inclusive society for everyone.

Psychological well-being and self-acceptance for a premature greying patient

Navigating premature greying requires a robust foundation of psychological well-being and self-acceptance. The journey towards embracing one's natural hair color prematurely involves various psychological aspects and coping mechanisms.

Firstly, fostering psychological well-being involves understanding and accepting the changes. This acceptance can be a gradual process, as the sudden appearance of grey hair can initially evoke shock, disbelief, or even distress. Acceptance doesn't imply immediate approval but rather acknowledging the reality and working towards embracing it.
Self-acceptance plays a pivotal role in this process. It involves embracing oneself holistically, beyond physical attributes. For individuals with premature greying, self-acceptance means recognizing that hair color doesn't define their worth or identity. It's about appreciating one's uniqueness and individuality, including their natural hair color.

Developing a positive self-image is crucial. This involves focusing on one's strengths, achievements, and character rather than fixating on physical appearance. Engaging in self-care practices, cultivating hobbies, nurturing relationships, and setting personal goals can contribute significantly to building self-worth and confidence.

Moreover, psychological well-being in the context of premature greying encompasses resilience-building strategies. This includes developing coping mechanisms to deal with societal perceptions, such as educating oneself about premature greying, seeking support from loved ones or support groups, and practicing mindfulness or meditation to manage stress.

Seeking professional help, such as therapy or counseling, can also aid in bolstering psychological well-being. Talking to a mental health professional can provide guidance and support in processing emotions, managing stress, and developing healthy coping strategies tailored to individual needs.

In conclusion, psychological well-being and self-acceptance are essential components of navigating premature greying. Embracing one's natural hair color prematurely involves a journey towards acceptance, self-appreciation, and resilience. By prioritizing psychological health and fostering self-acceptance, individuals can build a solid foundation for embracing their unique appearance and enhancing overall well-being.

Chapter 6

PERSONAL EXPERIENCES AND CASE STUDIES

Premature greying can be caused by genetics, stress, nutritional deficiencies, or underlying health conditions. While there's plenty of anecdotal evidence about premature greying, case studies often highlight individual experiences and their underlying causes. Consulting dermatologists or medical journals might provide detailed case studies or personal experiences related to premature greying and its management.

Stories from individuals experiencing premature greying

Amelia, a vibrant 25-year-old, noticed something peculiar in the mirror one morning. Amidst her chestnut hair were strands of silver. Initially dismissing it as a trick of the light, she soon realized that her hair was indeed turning prematurely grey.

Concerned, Amelia sought advice from a dermatologist, Dr. Bennett. Through their consultation, Dr. Bennett discovered that Amelia had a family history of premature greying, indicating a genetic predisposition. However, stress from her demanding job compounded the issue.

As Amelia grappled with this change, she met others with similar experiences through online support groups. Their stories varied—from managing emotions to exploring different hair care routines and seeking medical advice.

With Dr. Bennett's guidance and the support of her newfound community, Amelia focused on stress reduction techniques like yoga and meditation. She also adjusted her diet to include more nutrients beneficial for hair health.

Over time, Amelia learned to embrace her changing appearance. She found empowerment in her journey, inspiring others navigating premature greying to accept themselves and find confidence in their unique beauty.

This story aims to capture the emotional journey and coping mechanisms of someone experiencing premature greying, highlighting the importance of support and self-acceptance.

Story 2

James, a 30-year-old architect, was accustomed to the stress of meeting deadlines and managing projects. One day, while combing his dark hair, he spotted a cluster of silver strands. Shocked, he remembered his father had gone grey in his early thirties too.

Concerned about his appearance in a competitive industry, James sought advice from a trichologist, Dr. Lee. Through tests, Dr. Lee identified a combination of genetic predisposition and high-stress levels contributing to James' premature greying.

Navigating the professional world with greying hair became an unexpected challenge for James. His confidence waned, affecting his interactions with clients and colleagues. Struggling to accept this change, he isolated himself, fearing judgment and scrutiny.

Eventually, encouraged by a close friend, James joined a local support group for individuals experiencing premature greying. Sharing stories and strategies for acceptance became a turning point. He realized many faced similar challenges and found solace in their shared experiences.

Through Dr. Lee's guidance, stress management techniques, and the newfound support group, James began to regain his confidence. He explored different hairstyles and eventually embraced his changing appearance, understanding that his expertise and personality mattered more than his hair color.

James' journey taught him resilience and the power of community support. He became an advocate for self-acceptance, encouraging others facing premature greying to find strength in their uniqueness.

This narrative aims to depict the emotional struggles and eventual acceptance of premature greying, emphasizing the role of support systems in overcoming challenges related to self-acceptance. Insights into premature greying patient challenges, coping mechanisms, and acceptance

Premature greying can present unique challenges for individuals, affecting not just their appearance but also their emotional well-being. Exploring the challenges, coping mechanisms, and eventual acceptance within these individuals' journeys sheds light on a multifaceted experience.

Firstly, the onset of premature greying often catches individuals off guard, causing emotional distress. Societal norms and standards of beauty often emphasize youthful appearances, leading to feelings of insecurity, self-consciousness, and even a sense of premature aging. This can be particularly challenging for younger individuals who may struggle to reconcile their changing appearance with societal expectations.

Moreover, premature greying can evoke psychological distress, impacting self-esteem and confidence. The sudden alteration in one's physical appearance might lead to a loss of identity or a perceived loss of attractiveness, affecting interpersonal relationships and professional interactions. Individuals might also experience anxiety, depression, or feelings of isolation as they navigate this change.

Coping mechanisms for those dealing with premature greying vary but often involve a multifaceted approach. Seeking professional help, such as consulting dermatologists or trichologists, to understand the underlying causes can provide clarity and guidance. Managing stress through mindfulness practices, exercise, or seeking therapy can assist in reducing further hair discoloration caused by stress-induced factors.

Finding support networks, whether through friends, family, or online communities, plays a crucial role. Sharing experiences, exchanging tips, and realizing one is not alone in this experience can significantly alleviate the emotional burden. Additionally, exploring different hairstyles, using hair dyes, or embracing the natural grey can empower individuals to reclaim their appearance on their terms.

Acceptance of premature greying often marks a turning point in one's journey. It involves embracing the change, reframing perspectives, and focusing on aspects beyond physical appearance. It's about acknowledging that grey hair doesn't define one's worth or capabilities. Acceptance doesn't necessarily mean complacency; rather, it signifies embracing oneself wholly, including the changes that come with age or genetics.

In conclusion, the challenges posed by premature greying are not merely physical but deeply rooted in emotional and psychological aspects. Coping mechanisms and eventual acceptance involve a combination of self-awareness, seeking support, and reshaping perspectives. By fostering a culture of acceptance and celebrating individuality, we can create a more inclusive environment where premature greying is seen as a part of life's beautiful tapestry, not a source of distress or stigma.

Chapter 7

MOVING FORWARD

Dealing with premature greying can be challenging. Embrace it confidently or explore options like hair dyes or lifestyle changes. Consulting a trichologist provides insights tailored to your situation.

Future research and potential developments in managing premature greying

Managing premature greying has garnered attention in research. Future studies might delve into genetic factors, exploring targeted therapies to prevent or slow down greying. Understanding melanocyte biology could lead to innovative treatments. Lifestyle adjustments and stress management might also be focal points, given their potential influence on premature greying. As research progresses, a comprehensive approach combining genetics, biology, and lifestyle changes could pave the way for more effective management strategies.

Changing societal perspectives and beauty standards

The perception of premature greying within societal beauty standards has transformed in recent years.

Previously, grey hair was often associated with aging, and its premature onset was seen as a deviation from conventional youthfulness. However, contemporary society is challenging these norms and redefining beauty standards to be more inclusive.

There's a growing acknowledgment that premature greying is not a flaw but rather a natural occurrence influenced by genetic, environmental, and lifestyle factors. This shift is partly due to increased representation of individuals with grey hair in fashion, media, and advertising, breaking stereotypes and celebrating natural hair colors at any age.

Moreover, societal perspectives are evolving to appreciate the unique charm and elegance of grey hair. Many people now view it as a distinguished and stylish attribute rather than something to conceal or be ashamed of. This change is further facilitated by public figures and celebrities proudly embracing their grey hair, contributing to a broader acceptance of diverse beauty standards.

However, despite these positive changes, some remnants of the traditional beauty standards persist. Certain industries and societal perceptions still predominantly associate youthfulness with attractiveness, inadvertently contributing to the pressure on individuals with premature greying to cover it up or seek ways to reverse the process.

In conclusion, while there's progress in reshaping societal perspectives on premature greying, there's still a need for further advocacy and representation to fully embrace and celebrate natural hair colors, including grey. Promoting diverse beauty standards that appreciate the uniqueness of individuals, regardless of hair color or age, is pivotal for creating a more inclusive and accepting society.

www.ingramcontent.com/pod-product-compliance
Lightning Source LLC
Chambersburg PA
CBHW040739120726

48007CB00008B/145